D0048190

ISBN 978-0-9854190-3-5

Book design: Justin Carder and Alvaro Villanueva of Bookish Design

The Publisher wishes to thank Pete Danko, David Jordan,
Ron Tiongco, Jeff Kettmann, Nick Petrulakis, Karen Sweeney,
Jim Moorehead, Kim and Bruce Bochy, and Bookish Design
for their invaluable contributions to this project.

A
BOOK
OF WALKS

BY BRUCE BOCHY

WELLSTONE CENTER
IN THE REDWOODS

For my wife Kim

CONTENTS

A WALK WILL DO YOU GOOD

For millions of San Francisco Giants fans, it feels like Bruce Bochy is a member of the family. We're so used to seeing his face in the dugout, staring out at the field with a calm, unbothered look almost no matter what happens. He stares out at the action "with all the fuss and fury of a guy watching ribs slow-cook on the grill," as I put it in the April 2013 issue of *San Francisco Magazine*. This preternatural unflappability of Bochy's is essential both to his persona and to his development into probably the best field manager in baseball, a lock to end up in the Baseball Hall of Fame one day.

"He never looks like a guy who is beaten up by the job," ESPN anchor and reporter T.J. Quinn commented. "Even Joe Torre sometimes looked like he just came out of an alleyway beating. You could see the scars. With Bochy, you never do."

As fans watching at home we know he can't be as calm as he appears to be. We know that somewhere deep down he's as jumpy as we are when a Giants reliever loads the bases and goes 3–0 on a hitter with the game on the line. Yet time and again, Bochy has demonstrated that the higher the tension level ratchets up, the calmer he comes off, not just to us watching at home but to his players as well. They credit his even keel as a key factor in the Giants' unlikely run of winning the World Series in 2010, 2012 and 2014. His deep well of calm — "Zen-like equipoise" I dubbed it in that article — represents the ultimate vote of confidence in his players and encourages them, in turn, to take a longer view and avoid overreaction to short-term setbacks.

"One could make the case that he, not Phil Jackson, is the real Zen Master," Chris Ballard wrote in the December 18, 2014, issue of *Sports Illustrated*.

It turns out there are lessons to be learned from Bochy. We can't be him. Very few of us wear World Series rings or serve as a confidante to Buster Posey or Hunter

Pence. But we can be a little more like him. We can learn from his example. The Bochy Way is no great mystery. His approach is right there to be seen and emulated — or not:

- Be yourself
- Don't overthink
- Trust your people and trust your gut
- Lose yourself in a long walk

The last of these four points might be the key to the whole bunch. Yes, just being yourself is to a certain extent an art form one naturally embraces and pursues or not; it has to come from within, a calm and steady sense of who you are, so you don't constantly feel pulled this way and that. But in fact, we all need a little help sometimes in regaining our bearings. We all fall into the trap of reacting to events, caught up in this or that disappointment or setback, out of balance because we're not quite in the moment. Bochy's long walks help him catch up. They help him stand foursquare in the here and now. They help him jettison the mental clutter that builds up. They help him shoo away the remnants of any distractions so he can take life — and the ups and downs of a baseball game — as it comes, on its own terms.

"It's my time to kind of clear the head out," he says. "It's just a world of difference, it helps the mental side out so much, I'm convinced of it. I just think better after a walk."

Going for long walks carries over to the next two points as well. Bochy as manager understands a basic truth of life that we all know, but sometimes forget: *Most of our important thinking comes ahead of time.*

Bochy thinks every game through before-hand. Often he sequesters himself alone in his manager's office pregame for ten or twenty minutes and ponders the role he sees every player of his having that game. He'll mull emergency scenarios. He'll dream up enough surprise twists and turns in the plot line to fuel an Elmore Leonard novel. He'll study the stats, the matchups, and everything else he can to gain an analytic edge. Then he'll head out to the dugout and clear his thoughts and let the game steer his thinking. That is how he's ready to trust his gut: He knows what he knows.

"I watch the game," he told me. "You don't see me writing down a lot of things or having to look down at stats. They're important, but there are some things that you can't see on a spreadsheet. How a player is performing at that time, the confidence he's playing with. Or take it the other way: He's really going through a difficult time, and he's not comfortable at the plate or on the mound, or he's not quite there with his delivery. All these things, they play a part in any move that you make, and that's why you have to trust your gut, your instincts."

Bochy was taking long walks long before he moved to San Francisco to manage the Giants starting in 2007. The ritual of regular long walks got going in his San Diego years with his black lab Jessie, but the City by the Bay, ideal walking city that it is, with its sweeping vistas, its colorful people-watching, its rich mix of neighborhoods and landmarks, turned his walking into a fixture in his life. Often his wife, Kim, leads the way. "I'm a huge walker and San Francisco is the perfect city to walk in," she says. "So we're in the perfect spot for it.

I walk everywhere. I have a car but it sits in the garage. Sometimes it sits there until we have to go to the airport to pick someone up. Our son Greg, a firefighter, lives three miles away near Russian Hill and we walk over to see him." Their other son, Brett, is a pitcher in the Giants organization.

Another frequent walking companion is Brian Sabean, general manager of the Giants, architect of the three World Series championships in five seasons. But he's also happy to go solo. He'll go for brisk walks that are often like a run, planned in advance, or he'll dial it down a notch and walk wherever his feet tell him to go, whether that's a park or a corner pub, just so long as he's covering enough ground to feel like he went somewhere. Walking is a little adventure. It's a step through the Looking Glass into an alternate reality, knowing that when you come back you'll be the better for it. People in high-stress jobs like managing a big-league ball club are especially in need of the health benefits of regular long walks or other extended exercise — but everyone could benefit mightily as well from emulating Bochy and getting their steps in outdoors.

"That daily walking may improve mental well-being makes a certain amount of sense given that our brains and psyches are known to thrive on exercise," Bret Stetka wrote in a February 17, 2015, *Scientific American* article reporting on research demonstrating the physiological and psychic benefits of regular walks. "Regular physical activity has been linked with improved mood, enhanced creativity and a lower risk of depression. It can also improve symptoms in people with depression or anxiety. The rush of blood and oxygen to the brain that comes with working out also helps stave off cognitive decline, in part by inducing the growth of new neurons in the hippocampus, a brain region involved in memory and learning. In fact, exercise is one of the most effective means of preventing or delaying the onset of Alzheimer's disease."

Bochy's idea that good, long walks not only make him healthier, they make him smarter, has some interesting resonances. A host of scientific research supports the view, showing that regular walking can lead to more alertness, better problem-solving ability and improved mood. Research arrives every few months, it seems, offering additional proof of this basic truth, but it's hardly new. Friedrich Nietzsche and Henry David Thoreau, two giants of 19th century thought, were not only both ardent advocates of hours-long vigorous walks every day, both believed that walking improved their thinking. As Nietzsche put it: "Sit as little as possible; do not believe any idea that was not born in the open air and of free movement — in which the muscles do not also revel."

Basic health depends on being active — but that doesn't have to mean knocking yourself out with high-intensity workouts. In fact, a 2014 study by Lawrence Berkeley National Laboratory, Life Science Division, found that walking briskly was as effective as running in lowering your chances of having high blood pressure, high cholesterol or diabetes. "The findings don't surprise me at all," Russell Pate, Ph.D., a professor of exercise science in the Arnold School of Public Health at the University of South Carolina in Columbia, told the American Heart Association. "The findings are consistent with the American Heart Association's recommendations for physical activity in adults that we need thirty minutes of physical activity per day, at least 150 minutes of moderate activity per week or seventy-five minutes of vigorous activity per week to derive benefits."

Bochy found out for himself early in 2015 what a difference regular walking could make for his basic health. During his yearly physical examination at Giants spring-training camp in Scottsdale, Arizona, in February, irregularities with his heartbeat were detected. Team physician Robert Murray and trainer Dave Groeschner encouraged him to head over to the Scottsdale Healthcare Osborn Medical Center the following day — and, as he joked later, the next thing he knew, he's having two stents placed near his heart to improve blood flow.

Within days Bochy was back on the field managing the Giants, feeling better than he had in many months. He told the doctors about his penchant for regular long walks. They said without them he might not still be alive.

"There were two blockages, a little over 90 percent on two blockages," Bochy told me. "Once they put the two stents in, I felt so much better. I felt like I could walk up Camelback Mountain in Scottsdale."

One purpose of this book is to help people get to know Bruce Bochy a little better; he's become a beloved figure in the Bay Area and with good reason. But mostly Bochy is a vehicle: He's doing this book because he believes it's important for people to stay active, not just to get in their exercise but to have fun with it and to make the most of that exercise as an outlet that helps clear the mind and leads to a more balanced, relaxed approach to life. Of course that's not always easy to maintain! But it's worth taking the steps — you knew that one was coming — to give yourself a shot at feeling better and living better.

Bochy is donating the proceeds of this book to sponsor programs for young people at the Wellstone Center in the Redwoods near Santa Cruz, California, publishers of the book: specifically, our "Find Your Voice" weekend workshop for aspiring writers eighteen to twenty-one, and a weeklong Bruce Bochy Fellowship for young people looking to make a career out of writing about sports. For details on either, please visit the Wellstone Center in the Redwoods website at www.wellstoneredwoods.org or write Steve@wellstoneredwoods.org.

—*Steve Kettmann*

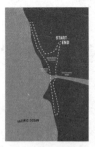

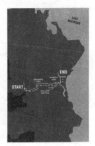

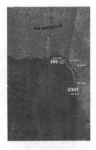

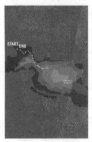

THE
WALKS

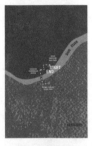

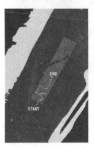

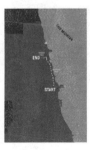

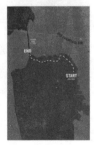

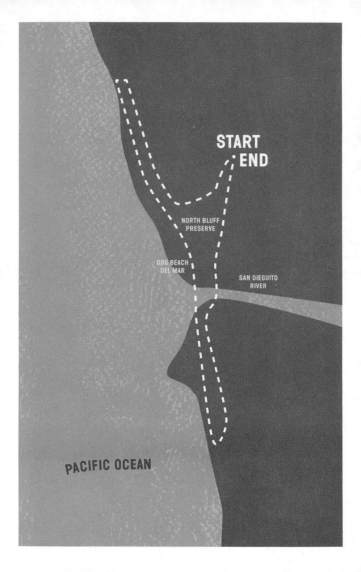

CHAPTER 1

TAKING MY DOG FOR A WALK

I still miss my black lab Jessie. We got her when she was a puppy, just six weeks old. We were living down near San Diego when I was managing the Padres and Elizabeth McNamara, a girl in the neighborhood, knew I wanted a lab puppy. I had two boys and I wanted them to grow up with a dog. Elizabeth was out in the countryside east of Poway, where we were living, when she saw a sign announcing that someone was looking to part ways with some lab puppies, actually they were three-quarters lab and one-quarter golden retriever. She called to tell us about those puppies, and it didn't take much urging. We hopped in my Ford Bronco and drove out there to take a look. You know how it is: Once you pick up a puppy, you're done. Jessie was part of the family after that.

That was really how I got into going for long walks. As a former catcher, I had to accept years ago that I could forget trying to do much running to stay fit as the years added up since my playing days. I'd go in for workouts whenever I could, maybe lift some weights and try to work up a sweat on the treadmill, but I can't say it was much fun. Jessie loved nothing more than being with me, and she needed her exercise. So it became our routine: I'd take her for long walks. She was my partner. We walked everywhere together all over Poway, which is about twenty miles north of San Diego up the 15. It's beautiful country, with rolling hills and great views and all kinds of different trails. Jessie and I explored just about every route there was to explore in the vicinity. She'd walk right near me and I'll tell you what, that dog never needed a leash. I remember one time someone from Animal Control stopped me about half a mile from my house in Poway and gave me a hard time. This Animal Control officer reminded me a lot of Barney Fife from *The Andy Griffith Show*. I thought he was going to arrest me for letting my dog run free.

"You've gotta get that dog on a leash," this officer told me.

The whole time, Jessie was just staring at him, like: *C'mon, give me a break! I don't need no leash!*

What did this guy think, I had a pit bull here? Jeez, that dog never got more than two feet away from me. I'd have a leash along with me, just in case I ran into a Barney Fife character, but usually I just had that in my hand. Another dog might approach us, or a whole group of dogs, and it didn't matter. Jessie would never leave my side. That was where she wanted to be.

Jessie couldn't wait for those walks. She'd bring her leash over to me, bless her heart, and drop it at my feet and wait for me. Dogs are just beautiful. They don't care if you win or lose. They don't care what's happening when you're not with them. They're always glad to see you. It's a great way to go through life. Jessie just enjoyed walking with me so much, and I took great pleasure out of watching how much she was enjoying herself. She just loved it.

That was a very special connection I felt with her when we'd be out for a walk. She'd look up at me and I always knew just what she was thinking or feeling. You can have somebody close to you and it doesn't have to be your wife, or another human, but your dog. I was thinking about her and what she wanted. She loved those walks for the feeling of freedom they gave her. If we were by a lake, it always made me smile to see her run and jump in the lake. It made you feel good that you were doing something that she loved, and of course you're getting benefit out of being there for a walk. It just gets you away from yourself to be out there walking with your dog. It clears your head. When you're done, you feel so much better. You get somewhat of a workout, but most important, mentally you get a break, and of course your dog is ready to lay down by you afterward and it's like she's telling you: *Thank you.*

I'd drive her over to the beach some days, which she loved, running along the sand and plunging into the surf. We were lucky, living in Poway, to have a popular dog beach less than twenty miles away, due west from us, next to where the San Dieguito River flows into the Pacific in Del Mar. That was an ideal spot for dogs, half a mile of beach for your dog to run around and play with other dogs. Technically it's known as North Beach, but everyone calls it Dog Beach — and it even earned a mention in *The Dog Lover's Companion to California.* "Dogs have so much fun here that they usually collapse in ecstatic exhaustion when they get back to the car," author Maria Goodavage writes.

Other times I'd take Jessie on camping

and fishing trips with me. People don't realize, but San Diego's got some country to it. I'd put Jessie in the Bronco and we'd drive away from the coast, picking up Highway 78 around Ramona and heading back into the wilderness there. You pass by Swartz Canyon County Park and once you drive past the little town of Santa Ysabel, known for Dudley's Bakery and Julian Apple Pie Factory, you're almost up into the mountains. There's a historic town there, Julian, that didn't have much more than about 1,500 people living there. I'd take Jessie and my boys up there and we'd go fishing and camping, sometimes at Cuyamaca Rancho State Park. We camped out there, right by the lake. I had a cattle rancher friend up in Santa Ysabel, Norm Feigel, whose family had moved to California from an Italian-speaking region of Switzerland. We'd go up and visit his ranch whenever we could. Jessie would run around his property and swim in the ponds, having the time of her life. Norm was a special friend, a man who lived an amazing life, working on the ranch starting at age five and serving as an Army medic in Okinawa after the war. He passed away in January 2015 and I sure do miss him.

I remember one time my wife and I took a three-week trip to Europe. We were there at the Louvre in Paris, looking at all this famous art, when we got a call from our son Greg, who was house-sitting the Poway house for us while we were gone. He was calling to alert us that a huge fire was raging in the area and we might lose the house. I was as concerned about Jessie as anything else, but Greg told me she was fine, if a little jumpy. The fire got so close, Greg was evacuated, and he did the best he could, grabbing some memorabilia and papers and whatnot and packing that into his car, along with Jessie, and heading a safe distance away to his home in Pacific Beach to wait out the fire. My wife, Kim, and I were going nuts over there in France, watching all these updates on CNN that made it look like the whole state of California was on fire. I'd call the house phone sometimes, just to hear the outgoing message on the machine. I figured if it was still playing, probably it hadn't been burned up just yet. We sure were distracted on that vacation. But when we got back, we found the fire had missed our street by a quarter-mile. Our house was fine. Jessie was fine. Soon we were taking our long walks again.

For more than ten years Jessie was my partner. Then one time when I was walking her she just stopped and looked up at me, like: *Hey, you know. I can't do this any more.* The next day, she wanted to try again, but we made it one block from the house and that was it. She was hurting too much to go farther than one block. That was the end of our walks. She held on until May 2010 — she was sixteen years old by then and had lived a great life. She never cared whether we won or lost, but I still think she'd have liked to be around later that year for the first of our Giants' World Series championships. As much as she loved walking with me, I bet ol' Jessie would have loved riding in the car with me during the victory parade through downtown San Francisco.

CHAPTER 2

BACK TO THE PFISTER IN MILWAUKEE
AFTER A TOUGH ROAD LOSS

It's well known in baseball that Milwaukee's Pfister Hotel, which first opened back in the 1890s, is haunted. I'm not going to tell you I've seen any ghosts there myself, because I haven't, but there are plenty of people who will tell you stories about seeing some crazy stuff there and I'm not about to call them liars. Pablo Sandoval refused to stay in the hotel with the team after an incident in 2009 when he said his iPod turned itself on and started playing music on its

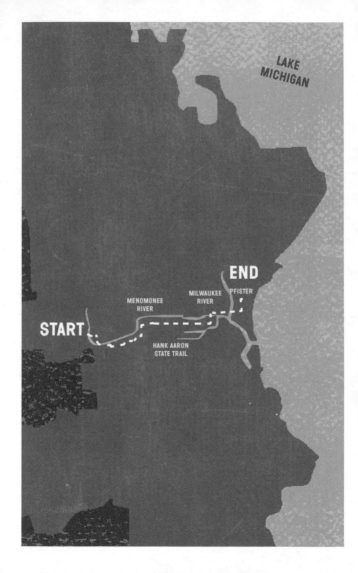

own — but he gave in after a while and decided he was going to stay there anyway. As for me, my scariest story relating to the Pfister is about making my way back to the hotel one time after a game.

This was June 2009, my third season managing the Giants. We came into Milwaukee for a three-game series and dropped the opener, 5–1, Matt Cain picking up only his second loss of the season to go with nine wins. On Saturday, Barry Zito had a shutout going through five and we put up some runs to take a 4–0 lead. But then Milwaukee tied it up in the sixth on homers from Prince Fielder and Casey McGehee and that's how it stood in the ninth inning, knotted up 4–4. Trevor Hoffman, who had been my closer for many years in San Diego, came out for the Brewers in the top of the ninth to face the top of our order and we strung together three singles and picked up a coupla runs on sac flies. You never assume a game is over until the umpire signals the last out, but with a two-run lead going into the bottom of the ninth, we liked our chances. Brian Wilson struck out Mike Rivera for the first out, then Craig Counsell legged out an infield single and Mat Gamel worked a walk to bring the winning run to the plate. I was finding it hard to watch by then. That was a win we had to have. But after two singles to tie it, Prince Fielder poked a game-winning double and it was one of those games where you just stared out at the field afterward, blinking, trying to hit the rewind button, because you can't quite believe it slipped away so fast. That was a tough one to swallow. I was still half in a trance when I talked to reporters after the game.

"When you have a chance to put a

dagger in them, you have to do it," I told them. "We've had a hard time doing that this season. That's as tough a game as you can have — especially after we got two off Trevor and then we couldn't close it out."

It's a funny thing. Over the course of the season there are certain losses that just stick in your craw. They bug you. You can't stop thinking about them. As a manager you fall into the old trap of second-guessing yourself, thinking through all your choices again, wondering if you'd missed something or forgotten to consider something. There's no avoiding that. It's part of the job. What you have to learn how to do is avoid second-guessing yourself about the second-guessing. You have to keep yourself from riding yourself for riding yourself. I knew I had my hands full with the challenge of getting past that loss in Milwaukee.

The team bus back to the Pfister had left and I was about to get a cab when I stopped myself. *You know what?* I said to myself. *The heck with that. I'm puttin' some shorts on and I'm gonna walk.*

They'd handed out meal money at the start of the road trip, like they always do, and I had that with me, around six hundred bucks in cash, but I wasn't thinking about money just then, I was thinking about the freedom to be alone with my thoughts for a while.

One thing all my favorite walks have in common is water. I don't know what it is. I just love walking along water. Maybe you do too. Coming out of the ballpark in Milwaukee, you head due east and right away you come to the Menomonee River flowing past. I crossed over the river, picked up the Hank Aaron State Trail and followed that along the far bank of the river all the way across town to the confluence with the Milwaukee River, just a few blocks from the Pfister, passing the Marquette University soccer fields and the Potawatomi Hotel & Casino along the way. But it was dark as I walked that evening and I really didn't see that much. I prefer to walk during the day, to take in the scenery.

Every city has its tougher neighborhoods, industrial areas with warehouses and sketchy characters here and there, and I felt like I walked through all of them that night. There I was, in my shorts and tennies, looking like a fish out of water in some of these placcs I walked through. I was getting some strange looks. Like: *Is he nuts? Or is he with the police?*

That was a long walk, more than four miles, but it felt a lot longer than four miles.

That's one I don't need to do again. I probably looked like I didn't have anything on me, wearing shorts and all, and of course nobody's going to recognize you — for one, it's dark, and two, I don't know how many baseball fans were in that area.

But you know what? I got back to the Pfister, went up to my room, and the last thing on my mind was that day's loss. I'd put it behind me and was focused 100 percent on going out the next day and getting a W back, which was what we did, too, breezing to a 7–0 victory. The night after that long walk, I slept like a baby — no bad dreams bothering me, no late-night worries about a game that got away, and no ghosts, either.

CHAPTER 3

MY WIFE AND I,
WALKING UP THE STEPS TO COIT TOWER

'll tell you something: I might have given up on taking regular long walks at one point or another if it wasn't for my wife, Kim, who keeps me honest. That woman is one hell of a walker! She and a couple of her friends walk together regularly and those gals move! I used to think that term "power walking" was a little bit of a joke, kind of good-natured exaggeration, but then I saw Kim with her friends out there motoring along and no question they put the

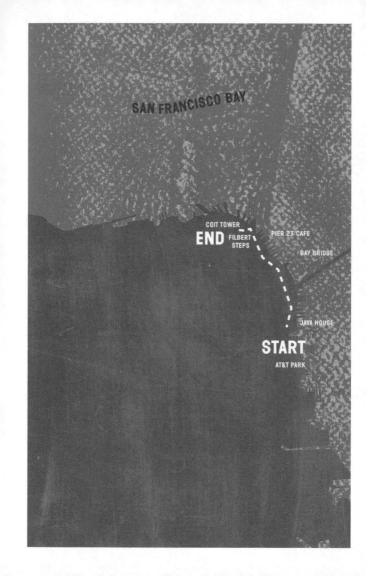

"power" in "walking." Kim and I often go for walks in San Francisco starting out at our condo across the street from AT&T Park, and one of our favorite routes is walking to Coit Tower and back.

Any walk starting at AT&T Park is a good walk. I know I'm a lucky man, I'm the first to tell you that. I'm happily married and the proud father of two grown boys I get along with great. But above all, I make a living doing what I love — and I get to do it in one of the most beautiful cities in the world. I've been to Rome. I've been to Paris, France. I've been a lot of places, and I'd put downtown San Francisco right up there with all of them for sheer breathtaking beauty, a place that makes you feel good just being alive.

The city has always been special, but it has also come a long way in the last couple decades. I remember when I was playing for the Astros and then the Padres, from 1978 to 1987. We'd come to town for a series against the Giants and we'd play our games at Candlestick Park, which was fine, a big concrete bowl like a lot of other big concrete bowls around baseball in those years, nothing special either way, down on windy Candlestick Point looking out on the whitecaps whipped up on the San Francisco Bay. The team hotel was up in the city and we'd go out after the game to get something to eat and downtown looked totally different back then. I remember going down to Fisherman's Wharf in those years and, let me tell you, it was nothing like it is now.

They'd built a structure called the Embarcadero Freeway in the 1950s that pretty well blocked out the view from that part of the city. Then after the Loma Prieta earthquake of 1989, the one that hit with the

A's and Giants gathered at Candlestick for Game 3 of the World Series, the Embarcadero Freeway had to come down and suddenly that area was restored with stunning views in every direction. By the time the Giants opened their new downtown ballpark, what we now call AT&T Park, that whole area along the waterfront had been redeveloped with countless different places to stop in to grab a bite with a view out on the bay toward Treasure Island and the East Bay in the distance.

Now when Kim and I lace up our sneakers and head out our front door, we walk a ways up King Street and we hit South Beach Park with its view of hundreds of boats bobbing in place at South Beach Harbor, and walk past the Java House. It's a great old place that looks almost like a shack when you see it in the distance, and it has been in business flipping burgers for sailors and longshoremen and everyone else going all the way back to 1912. Baseball players have been stopping in almost that long and the great Joe DiMaggio, a San Francisco boy, used to frequent the place. Kim and I walk from there, across Herb Caen Way, named for the great *San Francisco Chronicle* columnist, past Pier 40 and Pier 38 and up out on the wide expanse of the Embarcadero. I tell you, no matter what month of the year, no matter the weather, the people you see out there are always in a good mood and you always get a lung full of clean salt air that leaves you refreshed and invigorated. Then we walk by another Java House, this one Red's Java House on Pier 30, which longtime *Chronicle* reporter Carl Nolte has called "the Chartres Cathedral of cheap eats," a fitting tag for a place that opened in the 1930s and made a name for itself as Franco's Lunch, offering sailors a breakfast special of a cheeseburger with a beer. I love getting to know the history of all these different places. It makes you feel more connected to the city.

From there you walk under the Bay Bridge, emerging on the other side to a great vista of San Francisco's North Beach and the wide expanse of the bay stretching out toward Berkeley in the distance. The Ferry Building has been restored in the years since the Embarcadero Freeway was demolished and cleared away, and it's now a beautiful place to stroll through and people-watch. Kim and I like to go there as often as we can on Tuesdays, Thursdays and Saturdays for the Ferry Plaza Farmer's Market. There's a restaurant in the Ferry Building called the Slanted Door that started out as a little hole-in-the-wall kind of place in the Mission District, back when that was considered a sketchy part of town, until one night Mick Jagger stopped in for dinner — and liked it so much he stopped back again the next night. Soon it was one of the best known restaurants in town.

I love that walk along the Embarcadero so much, I could tell you about every pier, every stretch of the way, shoot, almost every crack in the pavement, I've done that walk so many times, and enjoy it so much, but if I described every detail for you here in my little book, I'd take some of the fun out of it for you. You've got to get out and take your own walks and experience for yourself all the sights and sounds and smells of that great walk along one edge of the city by the bay.

But I can tell you my favorite stop along

the way: the Pier 23 Café, known for its great seafood and for having live music every day. It's one of those places that was a dive for so long, it still feels like a dive, but in a good way. "We were a nightclub-bar-pickup-joint forever. We've kind of evolved into a San Francisco institution," current manager Mac Leibert told the *Chronicle* in 2013 in an article that went on to note: "In 1980, Herb Caen concluded: 'Place hasn't changed in 40 years.' It was a compliment."

Kim and I both love the place. We never sit inside, but always outside looking out on the bay. Especially on a sunny day, it just doesn't get any better than sitting there with that view eating a whole roasted Dungeness crab. We even saw some of the America's Cup from there. It's the kind of place where Kim and I can keep a low profile. We're there so often, we've almost become regulars. "We love seeing them in here," Mac says. "They just kind of relax out back and chill." That's what we do, all right!

From there Kim and I are liable to stick to the Embarcadero until just before Il Fornaio, an Italian restaurant we like, and from there hang a left onto Filbert Street, a wonderful little universe unto itself. It's one of the steepest streets in the Western Hemisphere in places. You pick that up from the Embarcadero after a walk through the plaza there and soon you're heading up the famous Filbert Steps, where locals tend private gardens you can enjoy on your way up. It's so steep, they had to put in steps instead of letting the road go through there.

The steps will take you right up to Telegraph Hill and the way up to Coit Tower, a San Francisco landmark as much as our beloved AT&T Park. I always love to dig around a little and learn the history, and I gotta say, the back story on Coit Tower is as good as it gets. The tower was built with money left behind by a grand lady of San Francisco by the name of Lillian Hitchcock Coit, who was a true eccentric in the best sense of the word, meaning she wasn't afraid to be herself, and also a huge fan and supporter of the city's brave firefighters. Lillie moved to the city with her family from the East Coast in 1851 and before long was dubbed "Firebelle Lil." I bet she was, too. She earned a reputation for loving to gamble with men, even if it meant dressing up as a man to do so. I'm told she enjoyed a good cigar and liked to wear pants back at a time when it was considered shocking for a lady to do that. She was friends with the Telegraph Hill firefighters from the time she was fifteen years old, was adopted as their "mascot," and even rode along with them from time to time.

When she died in 1929 she left behind a sizable fortune. Some of that money was used to build a statue of three firefighters in Washington Square Park and some to construct Coit Tower out of reinforced concrete in the early 1930s, providing a place with sweeping views of the city and the bay surrounding it, with Mount Tamalpais and Alcatraz Island as a backdrop. Kim and I love walking up the hill and passing by dozens of murals that were painted to go with the tower, murals that take you back through the decades and almost make you feel like you visited this place before, long ago.

Even though it was 90 degrees easy, clear with not a trace of fog, we weren't about to head home after visiting Coit Tower. So we kept on going, down the far side of the hill, and walked up Columbus Avenue until we found the perfect spot to grab some lunch there in the heart of North Beach. That's one of the great things about pushing yourself on a long walk: You always work up a great appetite, and food tastes even better. So does a bottle of beer. But once we had a meal in us and had a break from the heat, we walked over to Taylor Street — and Kim insisted that we ride one of those motorized cable cars on a tour of the city, right across the Golden Gate Bridge. Neither of us wanted that day to end.

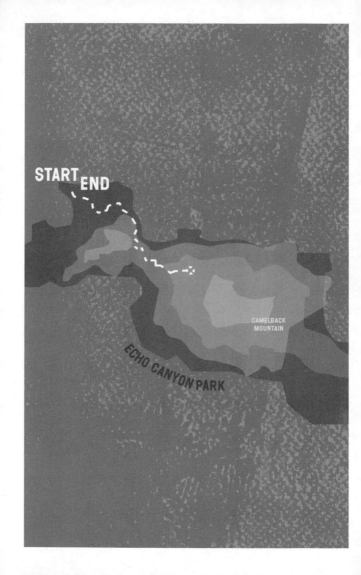

CHAPTER 4

CLIMBING CAMELBACK TO LOOK DOWN ON THE ARIZONA DESERT

If you're an old catcher like me, you've always got your aches and pains. Some days it's my left knee flaring up. Some days it's my left hip tweaking on me. In fact, some year before too long I'm going to have to have something done there, they've made so much progress with hip-replacement surgery. I have a lot of friends, many of them former baseball players, who've had hip replacement and they tell me they feel so much better and can move around way better. I'll be on blood thinners through the 2015 season, so I'm in no rush, but within a year or two I'll probably get that done. I tell you about some of my creaky parts not because I think anyone oughta feel sorry for me. Poor Boch! Oh no! But we all have our aches and pains, especially as we get up there a little in years, and yet you can't let that slow you down. You've got to get out there and walk anyway. Sometimes the walking will loosen you up and make you feel better. That's how it often is when I'm in Arizona for six weeks every spring. The dry desert climate is kind to the body, there's no two ways about it. I guess it's no mystery why so many snowbirds, as they're called, drive on down to the Southwest from Canada and the north every winter. The weather's perfect in Scottsdale for spring training. Once you get to summer, it gets just a little hot.

When I was a few years younger I used to walk to the ballpark in Scottsdale every day during spring training, put in my day of tossing BP and roaming around the infield and sizing up our young kids, then turn around and walk back home afterward. I enjoyed that route through the desert so much, I felt like I was missing out if I didn't walk it every chance I had. I'd head out from the place we rented near Indian Bend Road, up north near where the Diamondbacks have their spring training, off of North Pima Road. I'd follow Indian Bend to Hayden Road and cross the street there and turn south, passing the fairways of Scottsdale Silverado Golf Club and then cross over the Arizona Canal, a fifty-mile lifeline that dates back to the 1880s, and keep on Hayden all the way down. After Camelback Road you come to a golf course there, the Continental Golf Club, and I'd pick up a path there that would cut over to Osborne Road and right up to Scottsdale Stadium. Or I would cut across a couple streets at Miller Road, coming in the back way, and walk through the center-field entrance across from the Scottsdale courthouse.

I love spring training. All these years I've been going down to Arizona every spring and I love it more than ever. I like to get there early and get in some good walks before things get going. Once the games start, those are some long days for me, so taking long walks is my way of getting in a little exercise, instead of hiding myself away in a weight room or lumbering along on a treadmill staring straight ahead. Down in Arizona it's a crime to miss out on all that natural beauty spreading out for you in every direction. Those are some of the nicest looking sunsets you'll ever see and every night they're a little different, like walking along looking at paintings or something. The weather in the evening is ideal for walking and it's easy walking, not like there's a lot of hills or anything.

Mornings are also perfect for walking in the desert. If you want to take on the biggest hike in the area, climbing Camelback Mountain, usually you try to head over there early in the day when the desert heat is just starting to rise off the valley floor. Anyone who has spent time in the Phoenix area, even just driving through, knows the familiar outline of Camelback. What can you say? It's a mountain that has a hump, like a camel, that's where it got its name, and the hump is fun to climb.

In the spring of 2012, I decided to hike Camelback one morning with Karen Sweeney, the executive assistant to our general manager, Brian Sabean, and Dr. Kenneth Akizuki, our team orthopedic surgeon, along with Chrissy Yuen, who is medical administration coordinator and works with our trainer, Dave Groeschner. We had a night game later, which gave us plenty of time to make an easy outing of it, and we saw no need to get up at the crack of dawn. By nine we were heading up to the start of the trail, around back of Camelback, and we enjoyed the hike. First you set out on a series of big steps sweeping up the gradual slope of the mountain leading up from the parking lot, surrounded by the deep red of sedimentary sandstone, then the climbing gets more serious and you have to work your way around the side of the mountain. There is some steep climbing and soon you come to a hundred-foot-tall outcropping of red rock poking right up into the sky that really makes you stop and stare a minute. It's called the Praying Monk and it really does look like a monk tipped forward in prayer.

One of the features of a great walk is a lot of variety, and another is great sweeping vistas — and Camelback offers a ton of both. By the time you get up to the summit you're as tired from taking in so many stunning views as you are from all the climbing you've been doing. Well, almost. The doc and I were feeling pretty frisky and on the way down we really cut loose. We weren't running, not quite, but we were moving along pretty good. It's always exhilarating on the way down to cover ground in a hurry that took you a lot more time coming the other way, and you're moving so good, it's like the floor of the valley in the distance feels closer all the time. We got past the Praying Monk and were on the final stretch leading down to the parking lot when I heard my ankle go pop. I knew it was pretty bad. I'd rolled my ankle enough times to know that. But fortunately, I had a trained medical professional with me to give me an expert opinion.

"You need to put ice on it," Dr. Akizuki told me.

I stared at him for a minute.

"Twelve years of medical school and that's what I'm getting right now?" I said.

I had to hobble the rest of the way, or somewhere between a hop and a hobble, but at least we were near the end of the trail by the time the accident happened — and at least I was laughing. I had to put ice on it! I'd have never thought of that!

My ankle swelled up so much, we actually had to X-ray it, but it was just a bad sprain, nothing was broken in there. Even so, after that I was a little nervous about climbing

Camelback again. My left knee had always been my major problem, but I already had some history with my right ankle, too. Owing to a motorcycle accident I had a while back, that ankle is in bad shape. Ryan Klesko and I were shooting a commercial outside of San Diego back in early 2001 during my years managing the Padres, each of us riding big Indian Chiefs. We finished the commercial and I guess we got a little cocky and decided to just let 'er rip and have some fun.

I dropped behind Klesko and then did my best to catch up, flying around a corner at high speed to close the distance between us. Well, meanwhile, he'd stopped, thinking I'd stalled out. There he was when I came flying around that corner, walking his Chief to turn it around in the middle of the two-lane road. I had nowhere to go. I had no good options. All I could do was try to stop: I put everything into hitting the foot brake, too much probably. You should use the hand brake a little bit more, but I didn't have the experience to know that. So I slid right off the road. We were on the edge of a mountain and if I'd have veered off the road to the right, I'd have gone down about two hundred feet. I went to the left and went up the incline and turned my foot all the way around. The first doctor to look at it told me I had a compound fracture, but somehow it was just dislocated. Could have been worse! They patched me up, but I was in a boot for close to two months. In fact, we had Opening Day in San Francisco against the Giants and I was on crutches. Jon Miller was doing the introductions and when he read my name, he added, "Hustle up! Let's go!"

That was a short-lived deal for me, the motorcycle thing. I went and took a safety course, to do it right, but I never got to the point where I felt like I was riding with the wind, the way you kind of imagine. I was always a little nervous. If I would have gotten to where I was enjoying it, like I see with some of these guys, it would have been different. But once I got on the freeway it was white knuckles. Why ride if you're going to ride like that? One bad spill was enough for me. The tendon is off the bone of that ankle now. It flipped. So I don't have the support in that ankle I normally would have, which does tend to bark at me sometimes when I'm walking. I guess that's just an unfortunate thing about getting a little older. There's so much you want to do, but you've got to be smart about it. You've got to back off a little bit at times. But only a little bit. You can't back off all the way and stop being active, because that's why you're living.

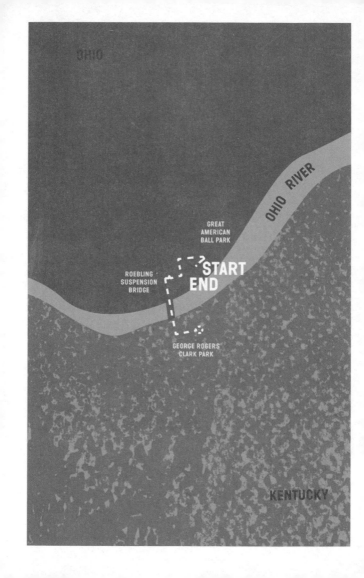

CHAPTER 5

WALKING FROM OHIO TO KENTUCKY AND BACK, OVER A HISTORIC SUSPENSION BRIDGE

I've said it before and I'll say it again: I love walking near water. Any city that has a river flowing through it probably has some good spots for walking, none better than a scenic bridge with a view up and down the river and right down into the current, if you want to peer over the edge. For me one of the highlights of coming to Cincinnati for a series against the Reds has always been the vantage point looking out over the Ohio River. For years the Reds played in Riverfront

Stadium, going all the way back to 1970, and then in 1996 they renamed it Cinergy Field. Finally in 2001 they opened a new ballyard, the Great American Ball Park. It doesn't matter much to me. Whatever they call their park, it's right there on the Ohio River practically spitting distance from the Roebling Suspension Bridge, which was the longest suspension bridge in the world when it was built in the 1850s and 1860s. Cincinnati's cool because you can walk across the bridge into Kentucky, walk around over on the other side, and then walk back across the Ohio River on the bridge and cross the state line again.

The first thing you notice walking out of the ballpark toward the Roebling Bridge is the sheer size of the massive towers at each end. They needed to be massive, to anchor each end of the suspension bridge, and massive they are, constructed out of a combination of oak beams and a monumental assemblage of limestone and sandstone. Every time I walk that way I have to kind of stare up at the tower on the Ohio side, struck once again by how huge it is. The designer of the bridge, an engineer named John Roebling, wanted to make sure the towers were more than massive enough to support as much weight as necessary as horses and people crossed over the bridge, so the towers were intentionally built to be oversized.

I got kind of interested in the designer, Roebling, as I walked across the bridge and read a plaque there that tells you a little about him. He started work on the bridge in 1856, but construction was interrupted during the years of the Civil War, starting in 1861, and it didn't open until 1866. Roebling was from Germany, which is where Kim's father's family comes from. Later on I heard that Roebling studied bridge design in Berlin and also studied with Hegel, the philosopher, but decided to come to the New World to seek his fortune. Roebling started producing his own high-quality wire rope, which he used for the suspension bridges he built, and after he finished in Ohio, he soon went to work on his master project, the Brooklyn Bridge in New York. He designed that famous span, but died during the construction, following a freak accident, but his son oversaw its completion.

When I look at the Roebling Bridge on the Ohio, I try to imagine the tools they had at their disposal back then, and I think: *How did Roebling get that bridge built?* It's incredible. We have issues trying to build a ballpark today, and they built this thing back when they did and it's as solid as any bridge anywhere today. You look at water lines on the bridge and see how high the water has risen during floods, and yet that bridge is still standing, looking unmovable. That's what I'm fascinated about, because they didn't have the equipment and techniques that we have developed over the years. It's like when I went to Rome and looked at the Coliseum. How in the heck did they build this back then? It's amazing to think of spectator sports, all those centuries ago, and to think when I'm managing the Giants, out there in front of tens of thousands of fans, that being in an arena packed with people is basic and it's something that goes way back. That's where the spectacle of sports started, back with a competition between gladiators inside the Coliseum. That amazes me.

Whenever I'm out for a walk as a visitor in a city, I'm always on the lookout for anything that will get me thinking about history. Once I walk across the Roebling Suspension Bridge and arrive in Covington, Kentucky, I like to take a left and follow Riverside Drive, heading north now. I check in on George Rogers Clark Park, which is best known for its views out on the river, but I like it for the seven bronze statues there. There's one of Roebling, looking dashing in a topcoat; and also of Mary Greene, who became a steamboat pilot on the Ohio and Mississippi rivers starting in the 1890s, a rarity for a woman; and John James Audubon, the naturalist and painter, who lived in Kentucky for many years (who knew?) and loved to go on long walks as much as I do. I like to linger around those statues, trying to picture myself sharing a little conversation with people like Audubon and Mary Greene and Roebling, but then I move on.

Of course, if you're a Giants fan, you know I'm including a chapter on Cincinnati partly because that city will always kick up fond associations for us. When we boarded a charter from San Francisco Airport to fly to Cincinnati in October 2012 during the National League Division Series, I'm not gonna lie: That was not the cheeriest of flights. It wasn't quiet, but it wasn't loud either. It was really business as usual. The guys were loose. We'd been smoked by the Reds on back-to-back nights, right there in our home ballpark, losing 5–2 and (it almost hurts me to type this) 9–0. We had no answer for Bronson Arroyo and he just mowed down our hitters like he could do it all night long. We were behind two-games-to-zip and no team had ever come back to win an NLDS after falling behind 2–0 at home. I tried to keep on an even keel, the way I always do, but it seemed a tall order to return the favor and swipe not just two games in a row, but three, on the Reds' home turf. Still, with a group of guys like that, you always believe and I had no trouble at all cranking it up for a pep talk before Game 3. That went over pretty well, but it turned out I was just the opening act. Next up was Hunter Pence, rallying the troops as only he can. It was something!

The crazy part was, we almost felt that winning was inevitable once we got past Game 3 of the series, an extra-inning thriller we won in the 10th inning when Buster and Hunter got us going. The Reds gave us an opening. Buster and Hunter moved over on a passed ball and then Buster scored when sure-handed Scott Rolen bobbled the ball.

Sometimes when you win a big game like that based on the other team's miscues, it turns the dynamic of the series even more. It sure did feel that way. Angel Pagan's leadoff homer in Game 4 gave us a lift right from the get-go, even though the Reds tied it in the bottom of the first. Barry Zito settled down and did a nice job for us and we had a 5–2 lead by the fifth and won going away. I guess for Giants fans it's like a tune you know so well, you can all sing along: In Game 5, we were locked in a pitcher's duel, Matt Cain and Mat Latos both putting up goose eggs, and then in the sixth Buster hit that grand slam we'll all remember to the end of our days, jump-starting us to a six-run inning, and we held on to win 6–4.

I tell ya, that one felt good. I was so proud of my guys for letting the game come to them and being ready to pounce on every opportunity. We had ourselves a heck of a good celebration that night, and the next day, we were kind of stuck in limbo, with nothing to do but enjoy what we'd done a little longer. The other NLDS also went to five games, and we had to wait a day to see whether the Nationals could beat the Cardinals at home to take the series. It didn't make much sense to fly to another city until we knew where to fly! We had a free day, so I did what I loved to do: I went walking. And kept walking. And walked some more. Kim was there, of course, and she and I had a day we'll never forget. The weather was perfect and we walked along those winding paths by the river, and stopped by and saw those statues I was mentioning earlier. Taking three in a row from the Reds was some feat, but afterward I needed nothing more than to decompress and that was what I did, walking here and there and everywhere, going back and forth from Ohio to Kentucky, taking in the day, being in the moment, and giving Kim my best "Life sure can be sweet!" smile. We didn't know what was coming next, but we knew we were excited about it. I felt refreshed and recharged, walking with my wife. Amazing what a good walk can do for you.

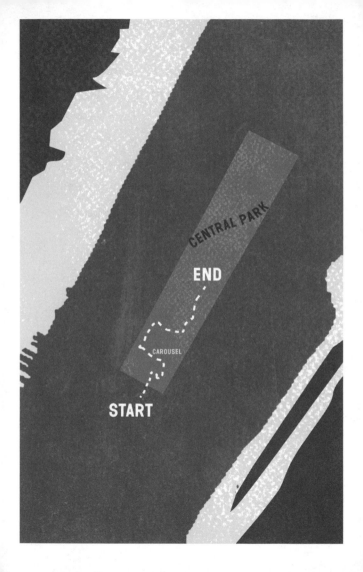

CHAPTER 6

IN NEW YORK MY WIFE AND I SPEND HOURS IN CENTRAL PARK

I f San Francisco is my idea of the best walk-ing city around, just for sheer beauty and variety, not to mention that great feeling of taking in a lung full of fresh sea air blow-ing in off the bay, I'd have to put New York right behind it. I'm not sure I'd want to walk through Manhattan every day. I might get a little tired of all the commotion. But for a few days at a time, especially when the weather is right, Kim and I just love our trips to New York. What a great city to walk in and take in the sites and the people. It's a little challenging, because you're running into so many people, it's so busy everywhere you turn, but at the same time you just can't beat walking as a way to get an experience of a city. It's funny. I tend to fall into a little bit of a routine at home in San Francisco with my walks. I have my favorite routes I take, like walking along the Embarcadero to the Pier 23 Café for crab and turning around and walking back, or climbing the steps up to Coit Tower, or doing the big one and walking all the way to the Golden Gate Bridge. But in New York I have a different mind-set. I like to let the walks take me where they will. We never go the same way twice.

Kim and I start out from the team hotel, just a few blocks south of Central Park South, and usually walk up Sixth Avenue toward the park. It kind of feels like home, in a way, we've made the walk so many times and enjoyed it so much. Even just walking through the city blocks, you see all kinds of places you know well from other visits. As you come up toward the intersection on 57th Street, you see the red awnings of Rue 57 lining the sidewalk and you know you're close to the park. You pass your little delis, your luggage shops, all of that stuff stays pretty much the same over the years. Then you come up to 59th Street, with the big blue banner pointing you to the Ritz Carlton Central Park looming off to your right, and the green of the trees opening up in front of you and yellow taxis all sprinting past you to try to get through that intersection before the light changes.

As soon as you cross the street and set foot in the park, it's like the atmosphere changes. You're still in Manhattan. You still feel all that activity and all those people and all that raw energy around you. But at least for visitors like Kim and me, Central Park always feels a little like a special kind of adventure. It's like a carnival in there. Right there on the corner you'll see horses and carriages stopping to pick up passengers, and next to them the pedicabs. Directly across from the Ritz is a giant statue of Simón Bolívar on his horse, which is pretty hard to miss. You can hit one of those little stands there for a hot dog or an ice cream or an iced tea, but I'm there to try to get in a good workout, so I'm not thinking about stopping. If I'm going to keep up with Kim, I've got to work at it, because she's a walker. In fact, when I'm off at the ballpark with the team, she'll keep right on walking most of the day.

"I love New York," she says. "There's so much to see. One time last year I left the hotel at one o'clock and didn't come back until nine. I walked across the whole park. I was in stores some of that time, but I didn't sit down for more than fifteen minutes the whole day."

Once Kim and I cross 59th Street, we generally walk right on up into the park through that area by the Pond. When Frederick Law Olmsted and Calvert Vaux were designing Central Park after winning a contest in 1858, they made a point of landscaping the area and surrounding the Pond with trees to help give you the feeling that you've plunged into the middle of the wilderness. What they called "the Promontory," now the Hallett Nature Sanctuary, wraps around the Pond and makes you think you've been swallowed up in some unknown woodlands. We keep moving and head past the Trump Ice Rink there, trying to imagine for a minute that it's wintertime, with snow on the trees and people sliding around on the ice in skates.

We walk past the rink there, picking up the long, gradual arc of East Drive, which takes you past a complex of buildings on the right, including the Central Park Zoo, and cut over on the 65th Street Transverse, heading back across the park now toward the Upper West Side. That takes us to the Central Park Carousel, which is always good for a smile. You hear that funny music sounding out, calliope they call it, even before you see the brightly painted horses. I always do enjoy a little history and I get a kick out of knowing that there has been a carousel there in the park dating back all the way to 1871. This is the fourth they've had, the last two having been destroyed by fire, and here's a good detail: The current carousel, originally built in 1908, was restored and brought over from Coney Island, where it had been left abandoned at an old trolley terminal. Our boys Greg and Brett are thirty-five and twenty-seven now and Kim took them on that carousel when they were small.

I said we like to be able to take a different path every time, and that's true, but there's a feeling of being pulled forward by the way in front of you, and sometimes we just keep going right along the edge of Sheep Meadow, maybe cutting across it a little, and walk up West Drive past Tavern on the Green with its big picture-glass windows. It starts to veer a little bit east as you get up toward Strawberry Fields, near the Dakota apartment building where John Lennon was shot, and we walk along Terrace Drive, past the Lake, to that area where they've got red brick all over the place and a whole bunch of steps leading down to the Bethesda Fountain, surrounded by a big round pool and topped off with an eight-foot bronze Angel of the Waters statue. Past there we're back on East Drive heading north through the park again, and that's an especially nice stretch. Over on the right is another pond where they have model sailboats and on the left is the Loeb Boathouse at the edge of the Lake. Then it's not far to the Metropolitan Museum of Art on the right, looking out on the Great Lawn to your left with its complex of softball fields, always a game going on there.

That's our basic walk, with variations, and it never gets old. I'll do that with Kim or sometimes I'll go out there on my own. In New York I'm usually focused on getting in a good workout, since everything in New York is a little intense and you want to make sure you have that release, but some days I'll say to myself: *You know what? This isn't going to be a power-walk thing, we're just going on a casual walk here. We're going to stop anyplace we want to stop.* On those days you're liable to find me anywhere. I'll keep on walking out the side of the park, down whatever street looks good to me that day, and if I see a little Irish pub along the way, which you always do walking around in New York, I might just duck in there and pull up a stool at the bar and order myself a beer. Those little Irish places are fun. Out on the street, in New York like in a lot of cities, there will be Giants fans and they'll call out, "Hey Boch." It's kind of amazing, how wide our fan base spreads. But most of the time in New York when I pop into a little neighborhood bar, they have no idea. We might talk about the weather or hunting or fishing or most anything. I'm just some guy stopping in to take a load off and rest my feet a little, cold beer in hand, a regular guy like anyone else. I like that.

CHAPTER 7

ON MY WAY TO THE IVY-COVERED WALLS: WALKING CHICAGO'S LAKEFRONT TRAIL

Sometimes I like to go for a long walk back to the team hotel after a game, the way I did in Milwaukee that time I mentioned, but if it's a great walking city, I might get ready for a game by walking *to* the ballpark. I find myself doing that a lot in Chicago, one of my favorite walking cities, where you can always count on dramatic backdrops and people-watching at its best. They call Chicago the City of Broad Shoul-

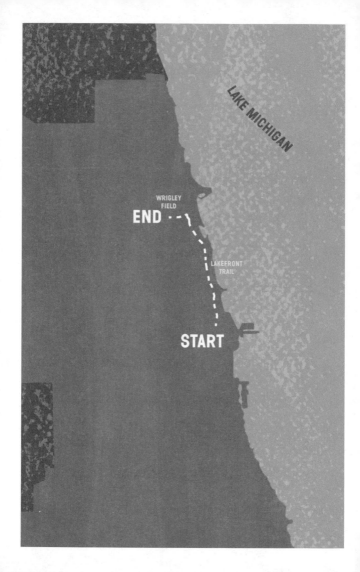

ders, or they do when they're not calling it the Windy City, that is. There's something down to earth about Chicago people you've got to like. Our team hotel is on the Near North Side near Water Tower Place, close to Michigan Avenue and the John Hancock building. If I have a little extra time, I can head south from the hotel for a great walk along Michigan Avenue through what they call the Magnificent Mile, full of shops and sidewalks stuffed with people, or I might follow the Chicago River toward the lake and walk out to the Navy Pier. But if I'm on the way to the game, then I walk north from the hotel.

You often feel a breeze coming in off Lake Michigan, which in summer helps cool you down. I walk up Michigan Avenue a couple blocks, passing the Drake Hotel, a snazzy place that opened in 1920 and soon became a local landmark. Most of the time when I'm walking, even walking alone, I don't want to have headphones on my ears, because I just love taking in my surroundings. I want to hear the sound of the water on Lake Michigan chopping in the wind. I want to hear birds squawking overhead. I want to hear the murmur of conversations in front of me that I couldn't understand even if I wanted to. That's part of the joy of walking for me, being focused on whatever I see along the way, alert to everything from a couple of songbirds making a bird bath out of a fountain to some friendly faces smiling at me from the far side of a picnic lunch. But I do love my music, especially country and country rock, and sometimes when I want a little kick to get me going, I'll crank up some tunes as I'm walking. It makes me move along a little faster, and it makes the time go quicker.

I'm a big fan of classic country, anything from Waylon Jennings and Willie Nelson to George Strait and George Jones. A good country song makes me smile because, well, it feels like home to me, losing myself in the rhythms of the music I grew up with. Funny thing, I was actually born in France when my Dad was stationed over there in Europe in the Army, and then the family moved to Columbia, South Carolina, and then on to the Canal Zone in Panama for a while. We spent time in Virginia before my Dad retired and we moved to Melbourne, Florida, which was where I graduated from high school and also spent two years attending Brevard Community College. That was where I met Kim. A good country song tells a story and if I'm out on a walk, that story will pull me right along just as surely as if I've got a wind at my back.

Take "The Gambler" by Kenny Rogers. That's one just about everyone knows, right? Everyone my age, for sure. That starts: *On a warm summer's eve / On a train bound for nowhere / I met up with the gambler …* Sure makes you want to listen to the rest of the story, doesn't it? Given that my job is a lot about being in the moment and being alert to whatever cues are out there during a game, I enjoy this part: *He said, "Son, I've made a life / Out of readin' people's faces / Knowin' what the cards were / By the way they held their eyes …"* From there it goes on to the famous part about knowing when to hold 'em, knowing when to fold 'em, and knowing when to walk away, which strikes me as some pretty good advice for baseball — and for life, too. "On the Road Again" by Willie Nelson is obviously a top choice, because it seems like we're always on the road again doing what we do. My favorite of all is Waylon Jennings, songs like "The Taker," "I Ain't Living Long Like This" and "Mammas Don't Let Your Babies Grow Up to Be Cowboys."

It can be fun, toddling up Michigan Avenue, which is as city as city gets, and listening to Waylon croon about how cowboys like old pool rooms and clear mountain mornings. In no time at all I've crossed over Lake Shore Drive to the Lakefront Trail, walking along the edge of the lake, and I'll say it again, I just love walking along water. It's at least a five-mile walk to where I'm going, so I keep a pretty good pace with not much time for dilly dallying. The Lakefront Trail is a wide, paved walkway that runs a total of eighteen miles there along Lake Michigan, all in the Chicago city limits, and I usually prefer to stick with it, rather than cutting up and over toward Wrigley Field on more of a beeline. On the pathway I walk right by North Avenue Beach on the right, with stand-up paddle board rentals and a place to eat called Castaways that has live music some of the time.

Up from there it's just about a perfect route for walking. The trail is flat and smooth, surrounded by sand, with beaches spreading out on your right, and beyond that a great view of the deep blue waters of the lake. You see all kinds of joggers and runners out there, people pushing strollers, but I'm happy doing my thing, walking along at my steady pace. When Kim and I walk that same route, we love the people-watching: You get all kinds out there! We also get a laugh out of seeing people spread their beach towels out anywhere they can, even on the concrete. She and I are both from Florida, so that seems pretty funny to us.

Kim and I walk awhile and turn back, but when I'm walking up to Wrigley Field I've got a ways to go. I pass by the boats in Diversey Harbor and over a little bridge, and by then I know I just have to reach the next harbor, Belmont Harbor, and I'm almost there. Once I get to Waveland Park, I take a left on Waveland Avenue and that's when the sense of excitement starts to kick in big-time. I don't think you can put on a baseball uniform and walk into a place like Wrigley Field, with its ivy-covered walls and echoes of history, and not feel some kind of shiver. The place was built in 1914 and back then it was called Weeghman Park, the home of the Chicago Whales of the Federal League. The Whales! The Federal League didn't last long and by 1916 the ballpark was hosting the home games of the Cubs. Managing there, where other managers have been leading their teams for a century now, always feels a little special. I've always loved coming into Wrigley for a series and seeing the way the local fans are enjoying themselves, whether they're gathering on the rooftop of one of the places along Waveland or fighting the crowds to squeeze through a turnstile in front.

One thing about Wrigley, though: In an old ballpark like that the visiting-team clubhouse is tiny. Once in a while you'd hear a complaint from one of our players, and that didn't sit too well with the longtime visiting clubhouse attendant, a real character named Tom Hellmann who everyone calls Otis.

"Wait a minute," Otis would tell anyone complaining. "It was good enough for Babe Ruth. It should be good enough for you."

You never hear much complaining after that.

CHAPTER 8

MY EVEREST:
TO THE GOLDEN GATE BRIDGE

Different walks are different. Sometimes you want nothing more than to head out for a walk you've done so many times, you know every turn and you don't have to pay any attention to where you're going. Those are walks to clear your head and unwind. You might mosey along at barely a stroll, if that's where your mood takes you. It really doesn't matter, so long as you're enjoying taking in your surroundings and letting your

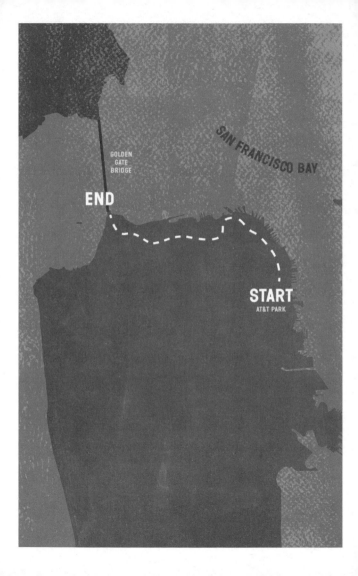

thoughts roll where they may. Other times you want a walk to feel like an accomplishment. You want it to be challenging enough to be good for conditioning and you want it to feel like an event. Not long after we moved to San Francisco for the 2007 season, back when I was still getting to know the city, I had one of those walks: I walked all the way from AT&T Park to the foot of the Golden Gate Bridge and partway back. That was a walk that was an event! I must have covered ten miles that day, but it felt like twenty, easy.

The notion of walking all the way to the Golden Gate Bridge was one of those ideas that came to me, and then I wanted to see if I could actually do it. Years ago a mountaineer was asked why he wanted to become the first to climb Mount Everest, and he answered, "Because it's there." I know what he meant. I guess anyone who is competitive enough to play in the big leagues, even as a backup in my case, has to have a fire inside that pushes you to do things. You don't tell yourself you *might* do something. You don't think *maybe* you'll get to your goal or destination. It kind of locks in place, all on its own, and you just know in your bones: I *am* going to make this happen. There's no drama about it. Quite the opposite, in fact. You just know and then you go out and live that experience.

That was how it was with my Golden Gate Bridge walk. I started out along the Embarcadero, the same route as Kim and I take on our way to Coit Tower, and that's where a walk gets to being a little like life: There's so much to see right in front of you, so much to take in and enjoy, you don't need to think about what's coming later on. Sure, maybe by the time you get three-quarters of the way there, your hip's going to feel like someone put it in a vice grip, or your ankle's going to make you want to curse Ryan Klesko ("Why couldn't you have moved that Chief out of the road a little sooner, buddy!?"), or you might wind up with the mother of all blisters on your toe. Those are thoughts for later. Right then you're on one thing and then another and another. You might stare across the bay at the outline of thirty-six giant white cranes all lined up together side by side at the Port of Oakland. You know what they are: They're out there to hoist huge shipping containers at one of the busiest ports in the U.S., but even knowing that, they sure do look like something out of *Star Wars*. You might find yourself transfixed for a minute by the visual of a boat cutting through the bay on its way back to McCovey Cove, making a neat little wake in the calm water that looks so much like a painting you have to shake your head, smile and look away. Or you might look down for a bit, just in front of where your steps are falling on the pavement, and let the rhythm of the walk lull you into something a lot like half-sleep.

Even if I don't stop for crab, I'm always going to follow the Embarcadero as far as the Pier 23 Café and maybe stop in and say hello to Mac. He's a good guy and always has something upbeat to say about the team. That's nice to hear! I won't lie! From there it all feels like you're flipping through postcards, the landmarks are so familiar. You pass the James R. Herman Cruise Terminal and see those big cruise ships out there looking like giant bathtubs painted white and as many other colors as they could get their hands on. That always makes me think of Kim: We went on our first cruise together on our honeymoon thirty-seven years ago, and love to sneak off on a cruise whenever we can find the time.

You pick it up a notch or two when you amble past the long lines waiting for the boats out to Alcatraz, and cruise by the Monterey Fish Market. Soon you're passing by that little park or square with neat green lawns looking out onto Pier 39 coming up on your right and vintage-painted street cars rolling along on your left. I understand people who get a little tired of seeing tourists everywhere, but I kind of like it. Aren't we all tourists somewhere sometime? They're usually friendly, and might even nod to me, like I'm some kind of local attraction, right up there with the sea lions barking out in the bay.

Past the boats of the Blue & Gold Fleet it's not far to Fisherman's Wharf, which brings back great memories for me, and then down past that row of restaurants along Jefferson Street that always makes me hungry, even if it's early and they're not opened up yet: Castagnola's, Lou's Fish Shack, Pompei's Grotto, then Cioppino's and Capurro's Restaurant. Then you're into Aquatic Park, where I'm always amazed to look and see whole groups of people swimming in the ice-cold waters of the bay. That's where I make my turn, going left to mix it up, and then it's through the Marina, where Giants fans are everywhere, and on into the Presidio for the last stretch heading out to Fort Point.

Talk about exhilarating! You see those two huge red-orange towers poking up out of the bay, the hallmarks of one of the most famous and recognizable bridges in the world, and you can't help but feel like one of the luckiest people in the world to be right there right then. I guess I've pretty well established myself as a little of a bridge nut. Well, the Roebling Bridge on the Ohio was the longest suspension bridge in the world for a while, and then it was the Golden Gate's turn. What a feat of engineering! That last stretch of walking, it's like there are giant magnets up there pulling you along and you don't think about anything except feeling good. The first time I did that walk, early on in my San Francisco years, I walked back to the Marina and had myself a nice breakfast at a place I liked on Chestnut Street called Bechelli's. (It's since closed, but they have Bechelli's Flower Market Café on Brannan Street not far from AT&T.) By the time I finished off my meal at Bechelli's and settled up, I was getting to feel a little stiff and didn't even think about walking any more. I caught a ride back home and looked out the window at all the same places I'd been walking by earlier.

That's a walk I recommend to everyone. If you need to move along at a pretty deliberate pace and stop often to rest, so what. Take the whole day! Make an adventure out of it. Whether you're a visitor to our city, or you've lived here your whole life, that's a walk that will make you feel good. It will make you feel alive. It will make you feel more like yourself. After that, every time you see a picture of the Golden Gate Bridge or you see it in a movie or out the window of the flight taking you somewhere else, you can kind of smile and remember what it felt like walking those last steps and being there at the foot of the bridge. I had a feeling I just wanted to walk to the Golden Gate. I thought it would be pretty cool. You know what? It was. It was very, very cool.

- -

WELLSTONE CENTER
IN THE REDWOODS

The Wellstone Center in the Redwoods, a writer's
retreat in Northern California, publishes books under
its Wellstone Books imprint. Founded by Sarah Ringler
and Steve Kettmann, WCR has been hailed in the *San
Jose Mercury News* and the *Santa Cruz Sentinel* as a
beautiful, inspiring environment that is "kind of like
heaven," and featured in *San Francisco Magazine*'s "Best
of the Bay" issue for its weekend writing workshops.
"Our focus is on helping create the writers of tomorrow
— and helping all of us unleash the writer within,"
Kettmann says. "We also offer writing residencies, host
book events, and welcome short-term visitors."

www.wellstoneredwoods.org